A Guide to Detoxification and Cleansing

Reclaim Your Healthy Body through Detoxifying

By: Katie Westengate

9781681279633

Publishers Notes

Disclaimer – Speedy Publishing LLC

This publication is intended to provide helpful and informative material. It is not intended to diagnose, treat, cure, or prevent any health problem or condition, nor is intended to replace the advice of a physician. No action should be taken solely on the contents of this book. Always consult your physician or qualified health-care professional on any matters regarding your health and before adopting any suggestions in this book or drawing inferences from it.

The author and publisher specifically disclaim all responsibility for any liability, loss or risk, personal or otherwise, which is incurred as a consequence, directly or indirectly, from the use or application of any contents of this book.

Any and all product names referenced within this book are the trademarks of their respective owners. None of these owners have sponsored, authorized, endorsed, or approved this book.

Always read all information provided by the manufacturers' product labels before using their products. The author and publisher are not responsible for claims made by manufacturers.

This book was originally printed before 2015. This is an adapted reprint by Speedy Publishing LLC with newly updated content designed to help readers with much more accurate and timely information and data.

Speedy Publishing LLC

40 E Main Street, Newark, Delaware, 19711

Contact Us: 1-888-248-4521

Website: http://www.speedypublishing.co

REPRINTED Paperback Edition: 9781681279633

Manufactured in the United States of America

Dedication

This book is dedicated to my friend Kris who is a big believer in healthy diet and lifestyle.

Table of Contents

CHAPTER 1- WHAT IS DETOXIFICATION AND WHY IT IS IMPORTANT

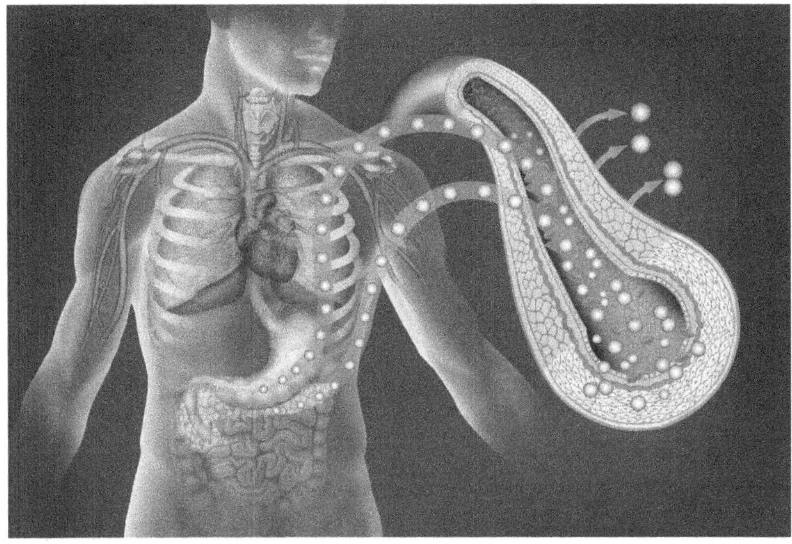

By now, you have most likely heard about body detoxification as it is very much in vogue, especially with celebrities. You might have wondered about the idea of colon cleansing and how it works. When you first hear about body detoxification, you may conjure up images in your mind that are unpleasant. Once you get to understand about body detoxification and how it works, however, you will have a different opinion.

Body detoxification concentrates on cleaning out your digestive system, usually by drinking a solution that is made to clear out your intestines and give the organs in your digestive system a boost. Although it may sound like a surgical procedure, body detoxification only involves drinking and then going to the bathroom. That is all there is to the procedure. It works to make sure that your digestive system is healthy.

When your digestive system is in good working order, your whole body sings. If your digestive system is not healthy, then your whole body suffers. In order to have a healthy body, you must have a healthy digestive system.

But your digestive system is the catch all for all of the toxins that you take into your body. Even if you are a healthy person who does not smoke, does not drink and eats only organic foods, you are still taking in toxins. They are in the air that you breathe, the water that you drink and…. Well, just about everywhere. These toxins linger in the body and find their way to the digestive system - a vital system that you need to maintain good health.

The digestive system is comprised of organs such as the liver, pancreas, kidneys and intestines. Foods usually enter the digestive system through the stomach and are then passed for processing through the digestive tract. Some foods and drinks that you take in making the kidneys and pancreas work overtime in processing them. All of the organs in the digestive system have a job to do in order to keep your body running healthy. Once food and drink is processed in the system, it is then eliminated by way of waste. Liquids are eliminated by urine and solid waste is eliminated through the intestines as feces.

In some cases, foods can end up getting stuck in the intestines. There are cases where people have had elements in their intestines for 10 years! In addition, the organs also take a beating when it comes to getting rid of toxins as well as some foods that can be difficult for these organs to process. Simple carbohydrates, for example, are very hard on the kidneys and pancreas as well as the liver as they tend to pass through quickly and make these organs work overtime.

Toxins in the air that you breathe enter the system through the circulatory system that brings blood to and from the organs. When you smoke, for example, the smoke is absorbed into your bloodstream and carried throughout your body. This negatively affects the digestive system. Even second hand smoke will take its toll.

Your skin is your biggest organ and when you take a bath or shower using chemicals as are featured in shampoo and soap, you are absorbing toxins into your skin. When you breathe in the air, you take the toxins into your lungs. It is impossible to live your life toxin free, although a good many people try. You are going to eventually go out and pick up germs that are in the air. It is inevitable that you will come into contact with toxins unless you decide to live your life in a plastic bubble.

Body detoxification clears the body of all of the toxins and foods that sit in the digestive system. Not only is it a good way to get the poisons out of your body, but it also works well when it comes to losing weight. Most people find that they can take off quite a few pounds simply by using body detoxification.

Drinking body detoxification fluid is similar to taking a barium enema, except you do not have to drink as much and it tastes much better. A barium enema completely clears out your intestines and is usually given to those who are having tests done on their colon or other digestive organs. This eliminates all of the waste from the body and makes you feel lighter. Not only can it get rid of toxins, but it can get rid of any waste that is lingering in your intestines.

Drinking the body detoxification formula is one of the first steps towards being healthier. You should also take proper precautions when it comes to your health and eat right, exercise and avoid bad habits. Body detoxification should be seen as a way to enhance your health, help you lose weight and keep your digestive system healthy. Good body detoxification will also fill your body with the nutrients that you may be lacking so that you stay healthy as well.

A Guide to Detoxification and Cleansing

Detoxification is a process by which you'll remove the toxic elements from your body in order to restore your health. Your body undergoes a lot of wear and tear throughout your day to day life. Toxins and free radicals are affecting your organs, your skin and your overall well being on the inside and on the outside.

During the course of your normal daily life, you could be exposed to harsh chemicals through your work environment. You could be ingesting harmful ingredients in your food. All of these elements working together can cause a very toxic environment in your body.

Things like cigarettes, acidic foods, caffeine, junk food and soda are all harmful to your health. If you are consuming these things on a consistent basis, you are harming your body on several levels. All of these elements build up in your system over time and can cause a whole host of problems including weight gain, memory problems and immune system issues.

Detoxification is a natural process that the body accomplishes all on its own under normal circumstances. However, when you have a poor diet and a stressful lifestyle your body isn't able to cleanse your system properly.

If your body is not able to do its job properly, you can take steps to help your body heal itself.

Detoxification can:

- Improve your immune system function

- Eliminate free radicals from your system

- Improve your ability to fight off cancer cells

- Cleans out congestion and mucous from your body

- Purify your blood

- Help you break your addiction to sugar, salt, alcohol and junk foods

Detoxification is slowly being acknowledged by modern medicine, but there are still skeptics out there. In this report, we'll go over the most popular detoxification products in addition to some more natural methods of detoxification that will help you lose weight and get the rest of the benefits of detoxification.

CHAPTER 2- WHO NEEDS DETOXIFICATION

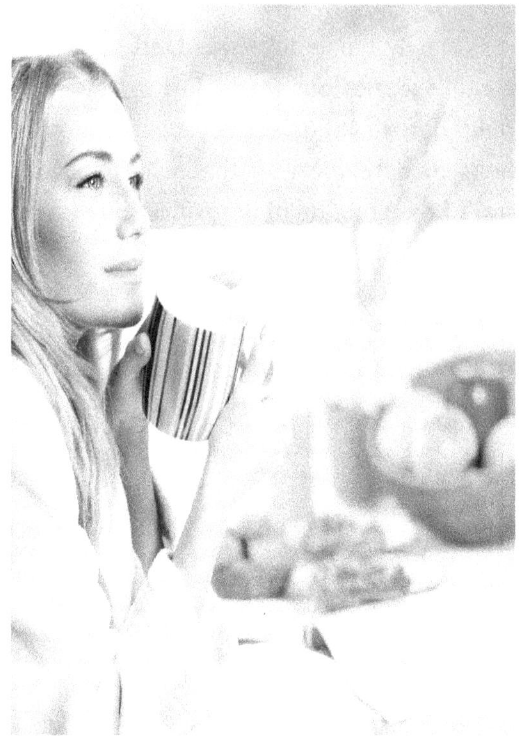

As stated earlier, just about anyone can make use of body detoxification. How often you use body detoxification materials depends on your lifestyle and the intent that you have for the body detoxification. If you want to lose weight, have a lifestyle that involves bad habits, such as smoking, you may want to use body detoxification more often. If you are just trying to maintain good digestive health, you can use body detoxification less often. But regardless of how often you decide to embark on this way to stay healthy, everyone needs body detoxification once in a while.

For Weight Loss

If you are trying to lose weight, you may want to try body detoxification. This will get rid of the waste in your body and you will feel much lighter. Many people who are looking for a way to lose weight opt for body detoxification. Body detoxification is one of the healthiest ways to lose weight.

Because you tend to store waste in your intestines, you may end up feeling bloated and retaining weight. Body detoxification eliminates the waste from your body and makes you feel lighter instantly. That being said, body detoxification is not a laxative. It is a natural way to eliminate waste from your system that leads to weight loss.

To Rid Yourself of Toxins

A lot of the celebrities are using body detoxification to rid themselves of toxins in which they imbibe on a regular basis. You can get rid of your body of toxins by using a body cleanse system. This will work towards keeping your body clean and free from the poisons that are in what you consume as well as what you breathe. If you smoke, drink or do not always eat a healthy diet, you can use body detoxification as a way to stay healthier and rid your body of toxins. While body detoxification should not be a substitute for practicing good health, it can help alleviate the problems that come with taking in toxins.

Just about everyone comes into contact with toxins. Ridding the body of toxins by using body detoxification is not only good for the digestive system, but also good for overall health.

Keeping the Digestive System Healthy

Remember, your digestive system and its health is vital to the overall health of your body. Colon cancer, which is cancer of the small intestine, is the number 3 cancer killer in the United States.

Colon cancer is the result of polyps in the colon. These polyps often result due to waste remaining in the colon. Body detoxification gets rid of the waste in the body and keeps the colon clean. On top of that, many body detoxification formulas have herbs, vitamins and minerals in them that can help the body detoxify the digestive system and can feed the organs with nutrients that are needed to keep it cleansed. A great many people use body detoxification as a way to maintain a healthy digestive system.

With natural body detoxification supplies, the body is fed a series of nutrients that not only end up helping the digestive system, but the rest of the body. The digestive organs send nutrients back through the body and to the heart, brain and other vital organs. Body detoxification cleanses the entire body through the digestive organs.

Passing Drug Testing

Those who get drug tested for jobs often using body detoxification at home to remove the remnants of illegal substances from the body, such as marijuana. While body detoxification does not help with a drug blood test, it can help someone pass a urine test for illegal substances or even tobacco. Someone who imbibes on the weekend can end up passing a drug test on Monday by using body detoxification.

While it is not recommended that you use body detoxification as a way to use drugs and pass drug tests, it can help you if you happen to make a bad decision and then have to take a drug test. A lapse in sense does not have to cost you your job if you use body detoxification solutions that are made for passing drug tests.

There are many different body detoxification products on the market. Most of them are made to maintain good health. Others concentrate on cleansing toxins from the body or as a way to lose weight. Anyone who wants to maintain good health as well as lose weight can benefit from body detoxification solutions and tablets that are sold on the market.

When you are body detoxification at home, you can even create your own solutions using natural ingredients to cleanse your body. Later in this book, we will discuss home remedies, how to use them and even give you some recipes on how to make your own at home body detoxification formula.

While everyone can benefit from using body detoxification at home, this should never be considered as a substitute for common sense when it comes to health. While body detoxification can help you lose weight, rid your body of toxins, keep your colon clean and even help you pass a drug test, the best way to stay healthy is to avoid toxins, drugs, and eating the wrong foods.

Losing weight can be difficult, especially if you want to take the pounds off fast. One way that you can use at home body detoxification is to help you lose those extra pounds. You can provide your body with nutrients and vitamins, it needs to function while at the same time, lose weight.

There are several solutions on the market as well as pills that can help you lose weight by body detoxification. The main ingredient that you need is water. You can use herbal supplements along with vitamins to help you lose weight with body detoxification. You can also use pre-made solutions that you purchase online or in health food stores as a body detoxification weight loss remedy.

Drinking plenty of water is one of the safest ways to lose weight. Water not only hydrates your system, but also fills you up and helps you expel excess water. You should drink 8 glasses of water a day, whether or not you are trying to lose weight. Water is even more essential when you are trying to lose weight.

Water alone, however, is not sufficient when it comes to losing weight. You need to supply your body with nutrients, especially if you are skipping meals. On top of that, you need to cleanse the digestive tract so that waste is eliminated. You should look for body detoxification supplements that will provide your body with the essential vitamins; it needs while helping you lose weight.

Body detoxification is the safe way to lose weight fast. Instead of taking weight loss pills that often contain illegal pharmaceutical ingredients, you can take off the weight with a body detoxification system. You can create your own body detoxification by mixing water with ingredients such as lemon and pepper that will cleanse out your system. There are also commercial brands of weight loss, body detoxification products that you can purchase.

Using the body detoxification systems to lose weight is safer than diet drinks that act as laxatives and contain chemicals. When you are looking for a body detoxification solution to help you lose weight, look for one that has all natural ingredients instead of one that is filled with chemicals as this will not only help you lose weight, but will also be healthier for your body.

Green tea is one of the key components when it comes to weight loss through body detoxification. Green tea acts like a diuretic and can help you lose weight quicker. You should drink green tea without sugar in order to get the effects. Drink plenty of green tea a day and you will find that you are taking off the pounds. Green tea can also be taken in tablet form if you dislike the taste.

Cranberry also works as a diuretic and can help you lose weight through body detoxification. Cranberry should be used in tablet form as the juice drinks that you purchase in the grocery store are loaded with sugar. Cranberry will also help clean out your urinary tract.

There are many kits on the market that you can use to create your own home body detoxification solutions that enable you to lose weight. These include those that are marketed under the name of colon cleansers. Colon cleansing is essential if you want to lose weight fast as it will eliminate any waste that is left in your intestines. This can help you lose weight at a dramatic speed if you use it often.

It is important that you drink plenty of water when you are body detoxification to lose weight. You never want to go on diet without supplementing yourself with water. By drinking 8 glasses of water a day and using a good, natural body detoxifier, you will take off weight quicker than dieting alone.

Of course, it goes without saying that you should exercise good common sense when you are trying to lose weight with body detoxification. Body detoxification is not a magic formula that lets you just lose weight while eating what you want. You still need to increase your activity as well as reduce the amount of calories that you are consuming. Body detoxification will, however, be an asset to your weight loss and will enable you to take in nutrients while cleansing your body of waste, helping you to lose weight.

CHAPTER 3- HOME DETOXIFICATION

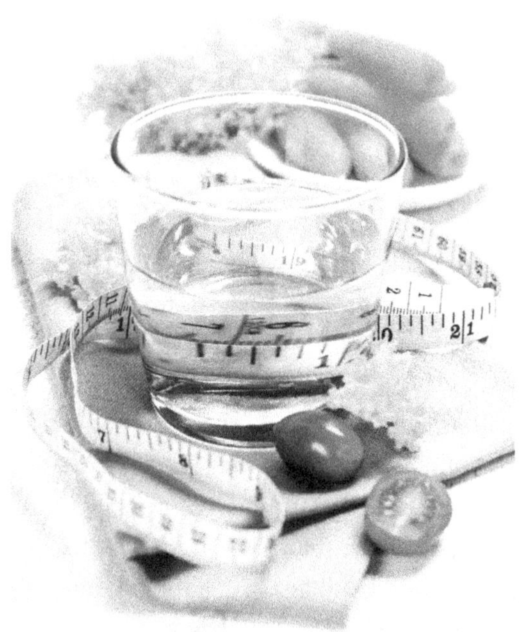

One of the primary reasons that people use home body detoxification is to detoxify their bodies. There are several products on the market that are made for body detoxification. These include products that range from those that can help you pass a drug test to those that can renew your body with organic herbs that rid your body of toxins that you may unwittingly take in.

Detoxification by body detoxification is usually done with a solution that you drink, although there are teas as well as tablets that you can take as well. Kits for home body detoxification often consist of tablets and teas as well as solutions that can be mixed in with water. It is often cheaper to buy these kits than to buy products that are already mixed together.

You should plan to use a body detoxifier to detoxify your body once a week if you have a lifestyle like most normal people that entails taking in toxins. You can mix up the remedy right at home and drink it. Most of the body detoxification kits that are sold online have pleasant taste to them and they will go to work right away to move through your system and ridding your body from toxins.

In addition to drinking the solution or taking the tablets, you will have to drink plenty of water. There are often instructions on how much water you should drink after you take the solution. Water will help the body detoxification product flush through your system and detoxify you.

Body detoxification not only rids your body of impurities that are found in the air, foods and drinks but it also can get rid your body of ailments. If you are trying to get over a cold, have stress or physical ailments, you will be surprised at how the body detoxification works to detoxify your system and make you feel better.

Choosing a home kit is the best option when you are seeking to body cleanse for health. This is not only the less expensive alternate, but it also allows you to use the kit whenever you feel the need to purify your body. The ingredients in the body detoxification kit should be all herbal ingredients that will work their way through your system and help you detoxify.

Drug Detox

If you are worried about passing a drug test, you can choose a body detoxification system that will cleanse any impurities from your body. This will work only if you are taking a urine drug test. There are several body detoxification agents that are on the market that will not only provide your body with nutrients, but will also color the urine so that it is not clear. The way that drug detox drinks work is that you drink them down and then follow them with several glasses of water. You have to do this a few hours before taking the drug test, although there are some that will work in less than an hour. After you drink several glasses of water in rapid succession, you will be able to take the test. Instead of your urine turning clear, as it would if you drink a lot of water at one time, it will have a yellowish tinge to it. The herbal remedies that are used in the drug detox body detoxification are not detectible by most drug tests.

No matter why you decide to detoxify yourself, you should be certain to use a body detoxification system that is all natural and does not contain any chemicals. Whether you use a tea, a tablet or a solution that is pre-made, you will feel good after you have cleansed your body in this way.

Colon Cleansing

A great many people who use body detoxification are interested in colon cleansing. These home body detoxification remedies can be used for eliminating constipation as well as making the colon healthy. Colon cleansing will eliminate any waste that you have in your body and clean it out.

Like the other body detoxification remedies, you can get colon cleansing in drink, tea or tablet form. There are also many kits that are used on the market for colon cleansing. Again, it is important to chase the solution or tablet with water so that it can make its way through your system.

There are various colon cleansing recipes and products that you can find on the internet. The ideal time to use colon cleansing is when you have time to relax and take the solution as well as have access to the bathroom. After colon cleansing works on you, you will feel lighter and more energetic. A great many people use colon cleansing as a way to lose weight as well. Most of the colon cleansing solutions is interchangeable with the weight loss solutions for body detoxification. They not only flush out the colon, but they also provide the body with treatment to keep the colon healthy.

There are many disease of the colon that can range from being inconvenient to being life threatening. One way to keep your colon healthy as well as maintain your weight is to use a colon cleanses body detoxification solution.

You can use a colon cleanse that you purchase at a health food store or online, or make your own. As is the case with all body detoxification, the key ingredient is water. In addition to water, you will want to add some natural products to help cleanse the colon and flush out the system. For colon cleansing, you should concentrate on using antioxidants that will not only help with colon cleansing, but will also help with health. One remedy that works well is pure grape juice mixed with water. This should not include the store bought grape juice, however, as it is filled with sugar. Resveratrol is also a supplement that can help with colon health as well as health of the entire digestive system. This is derived from the skin of red grapes. You can mix Resveratrol powder with water to make a colon cleanse that is healthy for colon health.

No matter what type of diet you consume, colon cleansing is a good way to keep the digestive system in good health. Whether you make your own solution or purchase a solution, you should use a colon cleanse once a week for good digestive health.

CHAPTER 4- NATURAL WAY OF BODY DETOXIFICATION

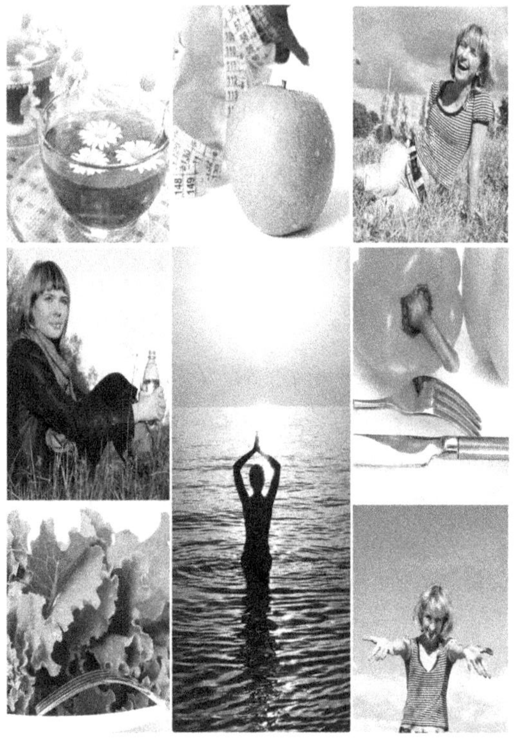

Although there are many products on the market for home body detoxification, you can also work towards cleansing your body at home without any products. One of the best ways to start body detoxification is to drink purified water. You should consume 6-8 glasses of water per day in order to maintain good health. Many people do not drink enough water and end up paying for it with weight gain and storing toxins in their body. Water is the natural way to flush toxins out of your body.

You can tell if you are drinking enough water by the color of your urine. If you are getting enough water, the urine should be nearly clear. If your urine is dark, it means that you are not drinking enough water. While it is more concentrated in the morning when you first go to the bathroom, it should get clearer throughout the day. Many people do not like drinking a lot of water throughout the day because they do not have time to use the bathroom frequently, however, it is one of the ways you can purify your body naturally. By keeping yourself hydrated, you will start to notice that you are better able to maintain your weight or even lose weight.

Another factor in natural body detoxification has to do with the foods that you eat. When you are trying to body cleanse, you should eat foods that are high in vitamins and minerals and low in fat. Eating at least seven fruits and vegetables a day will help you detoxify your system. Some of the foods that you will want to add to your diet include fish, blueberries, cranberries and leafy greens. These all work towards making you healthier by providing your body with nutrients that you need to maintain good health. You have most likely heard the old adage that you are what you eat. This is not just a saying, but a true fact. Start by cutting out fats, fast foods, sodium, processed foods and sweets from your diet that add toxins.

There is a large variety of organic products that you can choose as well. Organic foods are developed without toxins such as artificial hormones and chemicals. Eating organic foods is one way to keep your body clear of impurities.

Exercise is also essential for body detoxification. You should perform cardiovascular exercises that will work up a sweat as well as relaxing exercises, such as yoga, to eliminate stress. Many people today complain of stress over work, home or money. Stress can play havoc on your body and natural body detoxification should try to eliminate stress as much as possible. Exercise is a natural way to not only get in shape and burn calories, but also to sweat out toxins.

Supplements can also help you cleanse your body. You should take a good multivitamin in order to naturally cleanse your body. This will help you get the vitamins and minerals that you may be missing in your daily diet.

It stands to reason that you should practice good health habits and avoid behavior that leads to toxins entering your body. Do not smoke, take drugs or drink alcohol. These are habits that are detrimental to your health and should be avoided.

Once you get into the habit of naturally cleansing your body, you will find that it not only gets easier, but that you start to feel healthier and look better. Your entire body will respond to natural body detoxification. It is not difficult to use body detoxification at home once you understand how. When you start to see and feel the results, it even gets easier.

Chapter 5- Best Detox Drinks and Its Benefits

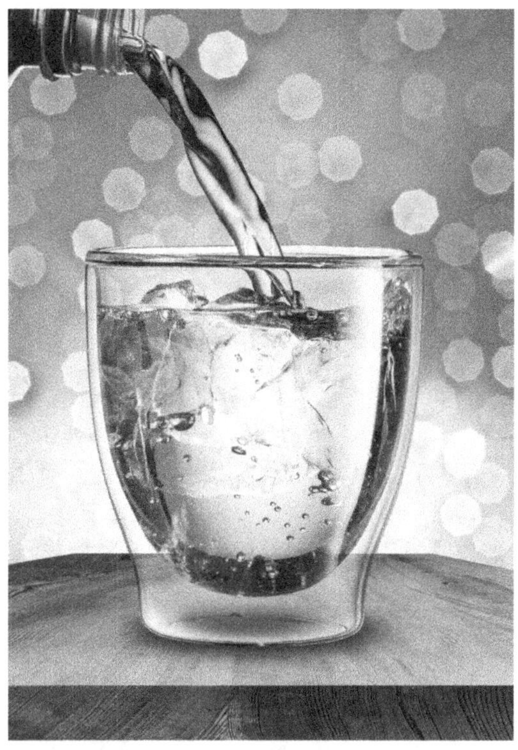

The best and the simplest detox drink that your body needs everyday is water. Ideally, we have to consume 6-8 glasses of water per day. To detoxify is to cleanse, and this process needs a lot of liquids to be present and flowing in the body in order for the detox organs to function well; the liver, lungs, kidneys, skin, and other detox organs function well and be able to do their job, which is to eradicate toxins from our system. This is why a lot of detox programs and cleansing diets are very particular on fluids. Some even disallow individuals from consuming any solid foods for a given period of time, surviving only on special juices for fasting or cleansing, most likely to allow the body to flush out remaining toxins. Like a well-oiled machine if your body has the right water level and keeping your body well-hydrated allows your detox organs to function well; the liver, lungs, kidneys, skin, and other detox organs would work well together.

Kinds of Drinking Water

There are different types of water, and you should know what kind of water to drink in order to stay healthy.

Tap water; most tap water systems are treated with chlorine, fluoride, and other chemicals which purify the water but are toxins themselves.

Distilled water or reversed osmosis water, have the particles and other chemicals removed, but the process also eliminates minerals in the water, and these minerals are essential to your health.

Natural and artesian spring waters are more accessible as they are sold in major stores, but these types of water are pricier. Generally, a home filter would work best in removing particles from your drinking water.

Common Detox Drinks

Lemon water – If you want flavored water, adding lemon is a great solution. In the morning, a cup of hot lemon water helps the body to burn more fat, stimulates digestion processes, and also helps in detox processes. Freshly-squeezed lemon juice and lemonade are also good for the body's natural cleansing processes.

Green tea – Green tea has been highly popular in recent years because of its supposed benefits particularly for weight loss. Green tea's most major benefit would be the high level of antioxidants it contains; these antioxidants are good for the liver, the body's main detox organ.

Green Detox Drink – Arguably one of the most popular detox drink recipes. In a blender, you will need to mix 3 kale leaves, 3 carrots, 2 celery stalks, 2 beets, 1 turnip, ½ bunches of spinach, ½ bunch parsley, ½ cabbage, ½ onion, and 2 garlic cloves. This is a very healthy cleansing drink; aside from the detox benefits, it is packed with other essential nutrients that the body needs.

Fruit Detox Drink – If the thought of drinking vegetables makes you turn green, perhaps this fruit detox recipe would be more to your liking. Rich in fiber, vitamins, and minerals, this drink is a blend of 4 oz. pure water, 8 oz. orange juice, ½ cup banana, strawberries or yogurt, ½-inch slice of ginger, 1 small garlic clove, 1 tablespoon flax oil, 1 tablespoon lecithin granules, 1 tablespoon freshly squeezed lemon juice (optional), and 1 tablespoon of protein powder.

Master Cleanse – This was made popular by Beyonce, who did the Master Cleanse diet for her role in Dreamgirls. This recipe requires warm water, 2 tbsp. of lemon juice, a pinch of Cayenne pepper, and 1 tbsp. of maple syrup. The drink in itself is designed for cleaning the liver and kidneys, but the Master Cleanse diet for weight loss takes it a step further by prohibiting all other solid food or beverage intake, with only this Master Cleanse drink to be administered several times a day (not recommended by nutritionists).

Other detox drinks of note include papaya drink (green papaya contains the enzyme papain which breaks down hardened toxins and removes parasites in the body); kiwi and grapefruit juice (abundant source of antioxidants, vitamin C, and fiber); and cranberry juice (promotes healthy digestion).

21 Benefits of Green Tea

1. Weight Loss

2. Fresh Breath

3. Reduces Cholesterol

4. Healthy Skin

5. Keeps Allergies at Bay

6. Healthy Hair

7. Managing Diabetes

8. Managing Blood Pressure

9. Prevention of platelet aggregation

10. Genital warts

11. Prevents Arthritis

12. Prevents Skin Cancer

13. Reduces Stress and Depression

14. Increases Immunity

15. Helps with Asthma

16. Healthy Liver

17. Prevents Osteoporosis

18. Cures Common Stomach Ailments

19. Natural Sunscreen

20. Stronger and Shinier Nails

21. Prevention and Treatment of Neurological Diseases

The Benefits of a Lemon Detox

1. Promotes Fresher Breath

2. Ensures balanced pH Levels in the Body

3. Improves digestive function

4. Strengthened immune system

12 Health Benefits of Organic Apple Cider Vinegar

1. Relief for rashes, stings and burns

2. Relief aching joints.

3. Battles yeast infections

4. Sore throat relief.

5. Helps upset stomach.

6. Useful in flu or chest congestion.

7. Sustains bone mass because it has magnesium, silicone and calcium.

8. Lower cholesterol and blood pressure.

9. Helps clear skin irritations, like acne and contact dermatitis.

10. Great for removing certain pesticides and bacteria from fresh produce.

11. Aids in weight loss studies show it increases metabolism, generates energy and reduces hunger.

12. Helps control blood sugar levels.

Aloe Vera Juice Benefits:

1. Cleanses toxic matter from the stomach, kidneys, spleen, bladder, liver, and is the most effective colon cleanser.

2. Healing and soothing properties for the relief of indigestion, stomach problems and even ulcers.

3. Help your body relieve tissue inflammation which often causes joint pain and even arthritis.

4. It strengthens the digestive tract, skin.

The Health Benefits of Cranberry Juice

1. Relieves inflammation of the bladder caused by bacterial infection or Cystitis.

2. Helps fight off heart disease.

3. Increases metabolism by converting fats into fuel.

4. Prevents Dental and Respiratory disease problems before they even start.

5. Detoxify your skin with the benefits of anti-oxidants, making it ideal if you suffer from acne or psoriasis.

6. Prevent kidney stones formation.

Benefits of ABC detox drinks

1. Prevent cancer cells to develop. It will restrain cancer cells to grow.

2. Prevent liver, kidney, pancreas disease and it can cure ulcer as well.

3. Strengthen the lung prevent heart attack and high blood pressure.

4. Strengthen the immune system.

5. Good for the eyesight, eliminate red and tired eyes or dry eyes.

6. Help to eliminate pain from physical training, muscle ache.

7. Detoxify, assist bowel movement, and eliminate constipation

8. Improve bad breath due to indigestion, throat infection.

9. Lessen menstrual pain

10. Assist Hay fever sufferer from hay fever attack.

Benefits of Water Detox

1. Lemon Water Detox. Lemon is beneficial in boosting your immune system as well as acidifying your urinary tract. This is a process of quickly and continuously getting rid of harmful substances out in your body system. Also, lemon regulates the digestive tract aiding your body to cleanse through regular bowel movement.

2. Lemon, Cucumber, and Mint Water Detox. Adding these three powerful antioxidants in your water creates a concoction of wellness. Lemon is an antioxidant, Cucumber is a rehydration plant, and Mint gives the taste a sweet sensation without the actual sugar guilt and relieves cramped up muscles.

3. Watermelon and Cucumber Water Detox. This tandem is also good for the liver since the watermelon contains the natural substance coralline that cleanses the liver from harmful ammonia by products. Cucumber is a complementary liver detox as well.

4. Lemon, Mint, Cucumber and Ginger Water Detox. Adding ginger to your water together with other detox fruits can give you a complete detox drink since ginger acts as intestinal soother and sweeps the intestines clean of harmful substances.

Chapter 6- Home Made Detox Drinks

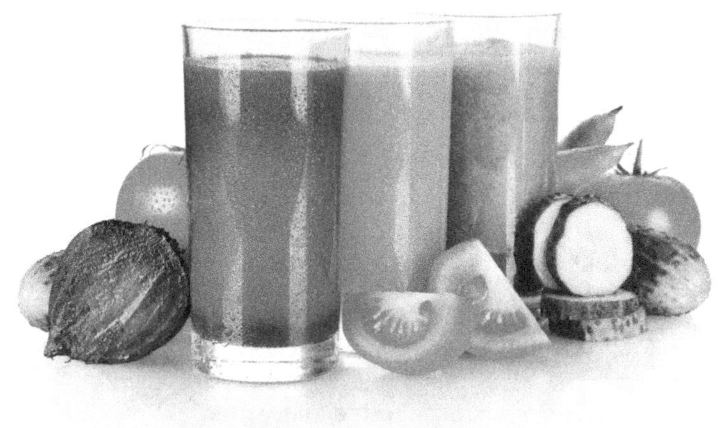

You can easily make your own home made remedies that are ideal for home body detoxification. This chapter will explore the different remedies that you can use and where you can get the ingredients for these body detoxification solutions.

For all of these homemade remedies, use only purified water. You can purchase purified water in the grocery store or get it right out of your tap if you have a water purifying system in your home. If you do not have a water purifying system, you should consider getting one for your home. This can help you keep your body free from some of the impurities you get from water.

Body Detoxifier One - Lemon Pepper Cleanser

Both lemon and pepper combined will work well to zip through the body as a cleanser. Lemon pepper cleanser is one of the easiest and effective home cleansing remedies.

8 Ounces of Water

2 Teaspoons of lemon zest

½ Teaspoon of black pepper

Combine the water and the other ingredients and drink it down. After you are finished drinking the solution, drink two 8 ounce glasses of water. This will help flush the solution into your system. Lemon pepper cleanser is good for the colon and entire digestive system.

For best results, use fresh ground black pepper and fresh lemon zest from a fresh lemon.

Alternate use - You can omit the black pepper and add one teaspoon of fresh lemon juice to the mix

Body Detoxifier Two - Italian body detoxifier

8 Ounces of Water

1 Teaspoon of flax seed oil

1 Teaspoon of Basil

1 Teaspoon of Oregano

½ Teaspoon of Garlic

Combine all of the ingredients with the water and drink it. After drinking, wait five minutes for the solution to settle and then drink two more glasses of water. This acts as a detoxifier for the entire body and is good for both the digestive system as well as the circulatory system.

For best results, use fresh herbs and garlic.

Alternate use - You can substitute Rosemary for Basil.

Body Detoxifier Three - Berry Detox

6 Ounces of Water

2 Ounces of Pure Acai Berry Juice

½ Cup Blueberries

4 Fresh Strawberries

Put all of the ingredients in the blender and mix them together. Drink them and follow the solution with an 8 ounce glass of purified water. This is a detoxifier that is loaded with antioxidants and purifiers.

For best results, use only fresh ingredients.

Alternate use - Substitute ½ cup of blueberries for the strawberries.

Body Detoxifier Four - Tropical Detox

1 Banana

1 cup unsweetened, plain yogurt

½ cup pure orange juice

½ cup pure pineapple juice

Put all ingredients into a blender and the mix them. This will be more like a shake than a traditional drink but works well to cleanse out the digestive tract as well as provide essential nutrients. This works slower than other body detoxifiers but is healthy for the colon as well as the heart and immune system.

For best results - Use only fresh ingredients and pure juices

Alternative - You can 1 cup of orange juice instead of half and half of pineapple juice and orange juice.

Body Detoxifier Five - Energizing Cleanse

8 Ounces of Water

1 Teaspoon of Maca Root

1 Teaspoon of Ginseng

1 Teaspoon of Acai powder

You may have to use pestle and mortar to break up the roots, especially if they are fresh, as they should be. You can purchase liquid Ginseng, although you are better off to purchase capsule forms. Grind up the dry ingredients, mix them with the Acai powder and then add them to the water. Drink down the mixture and then drink another glass of water.

This will not only give you energy to spare, but will also work towards detoxifying your digestive and circulatory system. If you are looking for a way to energize your body, this will do it.

You can purchase the supplements in any health food store or even online. Make sure that they are pure supplements and not just chemically reproduced. Ginseng is often available in "energy drinks" in stores - avoid that and get the actual product.

Body Detoxifier Six - Colon Cleanse Diet

8 Ounces of Water

1 Teaspoon of Flax Seed Oil

1 Teaspoon of FRESH ginger

1 Teaspoon of Grape seed oil

1 Package of green tea

This is a body detoxifier that works well as a colon cleanser. Add the ingredients together before adding to the water. You may need to use the mortar and pestle to grind up the ginger if you do not have a food processor. You want only to use fresh ginger for this cleanse. Open up the package of green tea and dump it into the mix.

Mix everything with the water and then drink. Follow it with two glasses of water. This is a good weight loss detoxifier that you can make right from products that you purchase at the supermarket.

For best results, Use only fresh ingredients that are pure

Alternate use - Use a green tea capsule and grind it up with the mortar and pestle.

Body Detoxifier Seven - Cinnamon Spice

1 cup of brewed green tea

1 teaspoon of honey

½ teaspoon of cinnamon

After you have brewed the green tea, add the cinnamon and the honey to the mixture and drink it hot. This is a pleasant tasting drink and will not only relax you, but will also cleanse out your body and help your heart.

For best results - Use fresh ground cinnamon

Body Detoxifier Eight - Kidney Cleansing

8 Ounces of Water

½ Cup pure cranberry juice

¼ Cup pure Acai juice

3 Teaspoons orange juice

Mix the ingredients together and add them to the water. Drink it down and then drink two more 8 ounce glasses of water. This will help clean out your urinary tract and clear up urinary tract infections.

For best results - Use only pure ingredients and 100 percent pure orange juice

Body Detoxifier Nine - Lavender Cleansing

8 Ounces of Water

1 Teaspoon of pure Lavender oil

1 Teaspoon of Flax Seed oil

Mix the oils with the water and drink. Consume another glass of water after to flush down the mixture. This is a total body cleanse and will detoxify all parts of your body.

Warning - Use only pure Lavender oil. Essential oils, with the exception of a few, are not made for ingestion Lavender oil is an exception, but it must be pure.

Body Detoxifier Ten - Tropical Delight

Ice Cubes made from purified water

½ Bananas

1 Teaspoon of Flax Seed Oil

½ Cup orange juice

¼ Cup Acai juice

2 Teaspoons of Lemon juice (pure)

Mix all of the ingredients together in a blender. Add enough ice cubes to fill the blender and then purifier. Drink the entire amount of the potion. This is a detoxifier for the body and can also substitute as a meal if you are trying to lose weight.

Body Detoxifier Eleven - Veggie Cleanser

1 Fresh Carrot, peeled

2 Crowns of Broccoli

1 Teaspoon of Omega Fish Oil

1 Teaspoon Flax Seed Oil

Ice Cubes

You need a food processor for this recipe, although it certainly cleans out the system and works wonders on the digestive system. You have to pulverize the vegetables so that they are like mush and then add the ice cubes and oils to the mix. Mix well and then consume the entire amount. Follow with a glass of purified water.

This is a safe and healthy drink that can be consumed on a healthy basis. It can also be used as a substitute for a meal if you are dieting.

Body Detoxifier Twelve - Vitamin Cleanser

1 Cup Green Tea - Hot

1 Capsule of Vitamin D

1 Capsule of Vitamin A

1 Capsule of Vitamin K

½ Teaspoon Cinnamon.

Grind up the capsules in a mortar and then add them to the hot tea so that they dissolve. Then add the cinnamon to the mix. Drink it down. This will add vitamins and nutrients to your body that you may be lacking. It is good for eliminating stress, depression and also healthy for the heart.

Green Tea Mango Pineapple Smoothie

1.25 tsp green tea

1 c frozen mango chunks

1 tbsp pineapple juice

1 c pineapple

1/2 to 1 cup water

Honey

Toss it all in a blender

Berries + Greens Shakes

1 cup frozen berries

1 to 2 loosely-packed cups of spinach

2 cups coconut milk

1 tablespoon coconut oil

2 heaping tablespoons plant-based protein powder

Directions: Blend until smooth.

Hemp seeds and Berries Shake

1 avocado

5 ounces frozen peaches

1 handful of raspberries

1 handful of hemp seeds

Unsweetened almond milk

2 dates

2 heaping tablespoons plant-based protein powder

Optional: 1 tablespoon ground flax seed

Directions: Blend and Enjoy.

Coconut Chai Shake

1 cup coconut milk (unsweetened)

1 tablespoon vanilla extract

1 teaspoon ginger

1 teaspoon cinnamon

A pinch of allspice

2 tablespoons almond or cashew butter

¼ cup shredded coconut

2 heaping tablespoons plant-based protein powder (ideally vanilla flavor)

Optional: 1 tablespoon ground flax seed

Directions: Blend until smooth and creamy.

Cashew Cream Smoothie

1 handful cashews

1 cup coconut water OR nut/rice/hemp seed milk of your choice

2 handfuls fresh mixed berries

1 ripe mango, pitted and diced

Optional: 1 tablespoon ground flax seed

Directions: Blend all ingredients together until creamy with a pinch of sea salt and enjoy!

Purple Haze Smoothie

6 ounces blackberries

2 cups of pineapple (fresh or frozen)

Water

Optional: 1 tablespoon ground flax seed

Directions: Put all ingredients in the blender and mix until smooth

Almond Butter and Jelly Shake

1 to 1½ cups almond milk

1 handful of frozen blueberries

1 to 2 tablespoons of almond or cashew butter

Optional: 1 tablespoon ground flax seed

 1 small handful of cherries, pitted a handful of ice

Directions: Blend until creamy.

Peaches and Cream Shake

1 cup frozen peaches

2 cups whole fat coconut milk

2 teaspoon pumpkin pie spice

1 teaspoon freshly grated ginger

2 heaping tablespoons plant-based protein powder

Optional: 1 tablespoon ground flax seed

Optional: Top with a few sprinkles of toasted (or raw) coconut for extra crunchy treat.

Directions: Blend until smooth and creamy.

Peach Apple Cobbler

¼ cup pecans (whole or crushed)

1 cup coconut water

2 apples, cored and sliced into chunks (if organic, leave the peel on for added fiber and nutrients)

1 cup frozen or fresh peaches

1 tablespoon fresh lemon juice

2 teaspoons vanilla powder or extract

1 teaspoon cinnamon

½ teaspoon ginger powder

Pinch of sea salt

Directions: Blend all ingredients together until creamy and enjoy

Spicy Green "Juice

2 big handfuls of spinach

About 1/4 cup parsley

Stalk celery, cut into chunks

1 small cucumber, peeled

1 inch piece of ginger, peeled

Juice of 1 lemon

6 ice cubes plus enough water to blend

Place all ingredients into a high-powered blender. Blend until everything is smooth and frothy.

All of the ingredients for these body detoxifiers can be found at your local grocery store or health food store. You need to make sure that you are purchasing pure ingredients and not those made from synthetics. You can buy a mortar and pestle online or in some drugstores and health food stores

CHAPTER 6- TIPS ON MAKING THE BEST DETOX DRINKS EVER

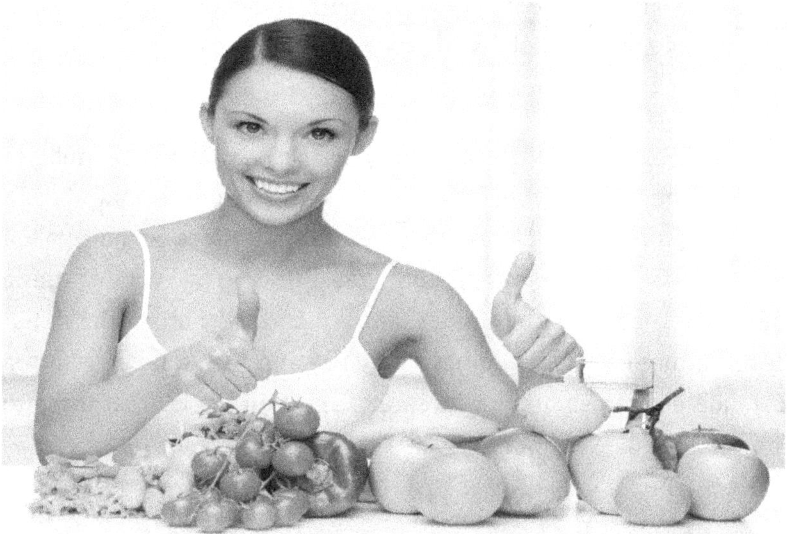

1. Change up the ingredients. Using different fruits and vegetables will help you get an even amount of nutrients and health benefits from the varying components. I try my best to use what's locally in season. If you're into green smoothies, be sure to rotate the greens every couple of weeks. This will also keep your smoothies new and exciting and prevent smoothie boredom.

2. Always use fresh fruit. The fresher the juice and ingredients you use in your smoothie, the better the flavor and nutrition. Use organic ingredients in your smoothie whenever possible, not only to increase nutrition and avoid pesticides, but also for better taste.

3. Juice it up. Juice your own fruits and vegetables for use as the base of your smoothie. Nothing is fresher, tastier, or healthier.

4. Spice it up. Various spices enhance both flavor and nutrition. Play with them and perfect the taste. Cinnamon, cayenne pepper, ginger, and nutmeg, are a few good options.

5. Seed it. Flax, hemp, and chia seeds are perfect for boosting the nutrition of your smoothies. Soak chia seeds in a little water to make a gel that gives your smoothie a nice smooth consistency.

6. Herbalicious. Adding Chinese herb powders like Ginseng, Astragalus and Rhodiola is a great way to increase the medicinal properties of your smoothie.

7. Healthy Tea Time. Use a healthy tea instead of water, milk, or juice as the base of your smoothie to boost the nutrition. Make a large pot of medicinal tea on weekend and store in half gallon mason jars for use during the week. If you're working on a particular health issue there's almost certainly an herb, if not several, that can help address that issue and would be a great tea candidate. Even something as simple as green tea is great place to start.

8. Make some Banana Cubes. Bananas are a staple smoothie ingredient, and if you like using frozen bananas in your smoothie, try this. Peel and break your ripe bananas into smaller chunks, and place those chunks into a big zip lock baggie or container before freezing.

9. Kid-Friendly Green Smoothies. Kids are picky eaters. Find something simple that they'll drink, then slowly over time work in the spinach and other greens.

10. Use coconut water ice cubes in your smoothies. Try coconut water ice cubes for flavor and additional nutrients including magnesium, potassium, and other electrolytes.

11. Super foods Galore. Experiment and try different super foods to really boost the nutrition of your smoothie. Maca, cacao, goji berries, bee pollen, aloe Vera, coconut oil, hemp seeds/protein, spirulina, and acai are great to start with.

12. Get Salty.Adding a high quality salt to your smoothie not only provides much needed minerals, but also perfects the taste. Celtic Sea salt is an excellent option.

13. Smoothie Sweetness. Using dates is a great way to sweeten your smoothie. Remove the pits and soak them overnight or for at least an hour before blending. If using a sweetener, stick to the good ones. Honey, maple syrup, and stevia are excellent choices. In the winter you might find your fruits are not as sweet as you'd like, causing your smoothies to not taste the best ever. Try using fruit juice as the base of your smoothie instead of water.

14. Healthy Fats. A good fat like coconut, flax, or hemp oil, an avocado, or cream will keep you satiated and full of energy for hours, and put the smooth in smoothie.

15. Milk and young coconut water deliver a probiotic punch while improving digestion and nutrient assimilation.

ABOUT THE AUTHOR

Katie Westengate became interested in healthy and natural remedies after the birth of her two daughters made her much more concerned about creating a healthy lifestyle for her family. Through research and experimentation, Katie has discovered some amazing recipes to help to improve overall health. Katie has worked hard to make available to help everyone get the vital information needed to maintain health in their busy lives.

www.ingramcontent.com/pod-product-compliance
Lightning Source LLC
Chambersburg PA
CBHW050706250726
48662CB00002B/875